Kettlebell Workout

A Total Body Workout Guide to Burn Fat, Lose Weight and Build Lean Muscle

RON KNESS

Contents

Disclaimer 1

Introduction... 2

Why Kettlebell Fitness Is Hot................................... 5

Top Kettlebell Exercises 8

Kettlebell Drills You Can Do at Home 13

Kettlebell Workout Tips 17

What to Expect in Kettlebell Classes..................... 22

Kettlebell for Women 25

Buying a Kettlebell.. 28

Top 5 Kettlebells Reviewed & Compared 35

How to Lose Weight With a Kettlebell 44

The Forgotten Muscle Groups That Kettlebell Training

Works... 47

Final Thoughts... 50

Other Relevant Books by This Author................... 53

About the Author 58

Disclaimer

This publication is for informational purposes only and is not intended as medical advice. Medical advice should always be obtained from a qualified medical professional for any health conditions or symptoms associated with them.
Every possible effort has been made in preparing and researching this material. We make no warranties with respect to the accuracy, applicability of its contents or any omissions.

See your healthcare professional before starting any diet, health or exercise program!

Introduction

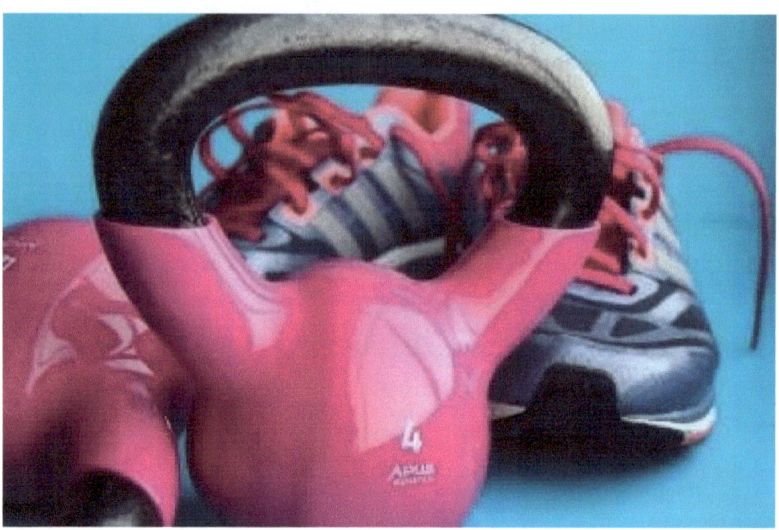

The kettlebell is traditionally a cast iron weight that originated in Russia and has now taken the fitness world by storm. It's a wonderful workout for both men and women of any age and at any degree of fitness.

This is the kind of workout where repetition is key to your success. You'll be working out in bursts with breaks in between to recover from the intense cycles of training. You'll find your breathing sometimes labored, unlike traditional weight training that's slower in pace.

Kettlebell workouts typically have you doing total body movements that are known by the following names: snatch, swing, high pull, and one known as the clean and jerk. The names may sound funny, but the effect they have on your fitness is amazing.

Kettlebell training helps you increase your strength, but it also improves your cardiovascular abilities because of the swinging motion you implement that isn't found when you use simple dumbbells in your workout routines.

When you start using kettlebells, you'll notice that your strength builds and your endurance expands beyond what you'd had before. You'll be performing moves with your kettlebell that affect your shoulders, back and legs – it's a total body workout!

Because it impacts your back, it's not a good workout to jump into if you currently suffer from back problems. But at the same time, it can strengthen the muscles in your back, so you may be able to start off with gentle movements and increase from there.

Some people liken the kettlebell to old fashioned medicine balls, but the variants they allow in training with the handles and movement options offer a better combination workout than simply catching a weight in your hands.

You'll be able to decide if you want to perform a grind or ballistic movement. Grinds are slow and calculated, emphasizing strength. Ballistic exercises are those where movement and speed play an important role.

The one thing you want to understand when you start using kettlebells is that it's important not to rush your abilities. These are heavy weights, and starting out with one that's too heavy for you can cause more harm than good if you injure yourself in the process.

Most people find kettlebell training to be one of the more fun activities they've tried. It's not as boring as walking on a treadmill or lifting a dumb bell. You will need room to swing and move, but the equipment itself doesn't take up a lot of space.

Why Kettlebell Fitness Is Hot

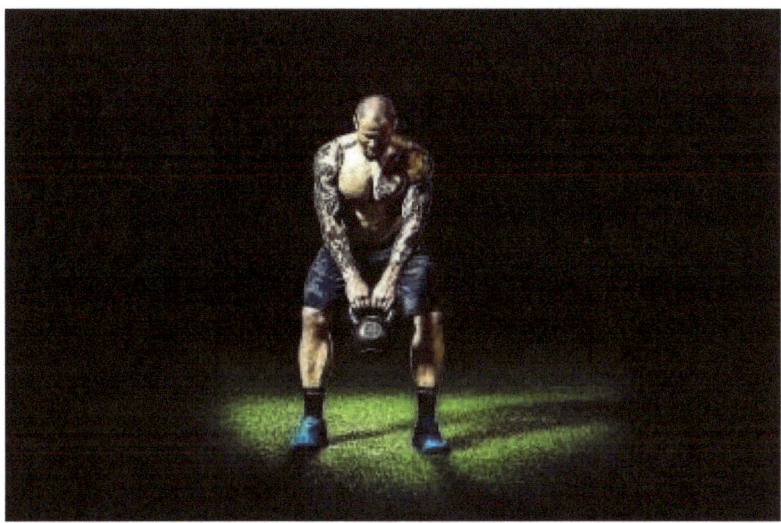

There are four primary reasons why you may have been hearing the buzzword "kettlebell" a lot lately. It's gone from a traditional form of exercise to a fitness craze both genders are passionate about.

The first reason why kettlebell fitness is hot is because weight loss continues to be an issue many people around the globe are striving to achieve. Being overweight is something affecting more people than ever before and weight-related diseases like diabetes are exploding.

Kettlebell fitness helps people lose weight because it does two things at once. It helps build strength with its elements of weight training. Plus, the fast movements in the ballistic exercises provide a form of cardiovascular exercise that help you burn fat faster. So it actually is a hybrid of cardio and strength training.

Many kettlebell classes will have a primary focus of fat loss and conditioning, so the training is fast-paced and geared toward those who want to sweat a lot and see results faster.

Another reason why kettlebell fitness is hot is that it's been proven to assist in aiding with back pain. Back pain is something that has few treatments short of medical surgery. When kettlebells are used, not only is the back repaired, but the neck, too.

Unfortunately, many people who suffer from back pain believe they have to avoid weight training. They're scared of kettlebells. But not only do they ease back pain – they prevent you from re-injuring yourself later, if you lift smart.

Kettlebell exercises help you gain more strength in your trunk and core, which is where you need the most strength for your back. The key is to train properly, so learning the fundamental moves is imperative to your success.

Busy moms and dads are another reason kettlebell fitness is a hot topic. Because the training is so intense, and usually includes a total body workout, you get more results with a shorter period of time.

This allows busy parents to work in their routine during the day in short bursts, rather than having to carve out a full hour to get the fitness benefits they desire. After participating in kettlebell training, moms and dads report to have a better quality of life.

Competitive athletes are also fueling the kettlebell fitness craze. Not only does it help them gain mass, stay lean, increase flexibility and enhance their endurance, but it helps rehabilitate them in the event that they're injured. Once trained, it prevents future injuries as well.

Kettlebell training helps them strengthen their abdominal muscles, legs, arms, back and core. Because the training requires great attention to form, it helps the athletes perform better, too.

Top Kettlebell Exercises

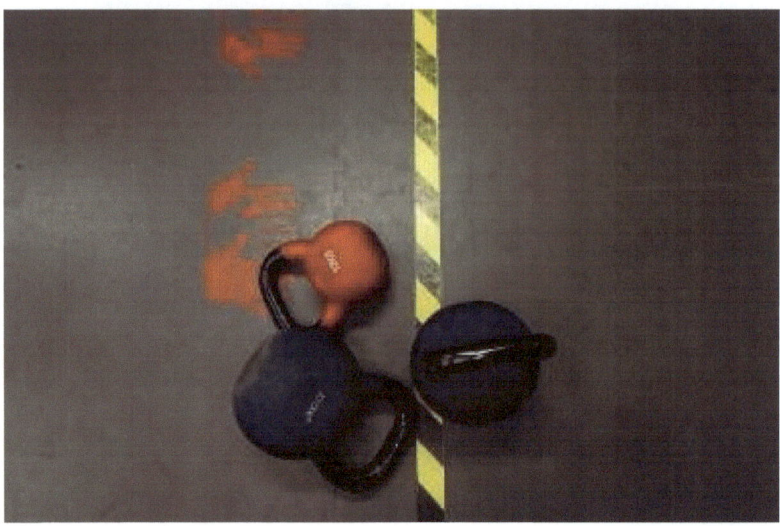

As mentioned earlier. you can break up your kettlebell exercises into the grinds and ballistics. You have to understand your grinds because they are the basic strategies for your ballistic movements.

Before you can start doing any of the kettlebell exercises, you first have to learn how to pick up a kettlebell from a dead lift position. Keep your back straight and your head up when you bend down to pick it up and don't use your back as the primary source of strength – use your legs instead.

Next, you can move on to your squats. There are different kinds of squats. A basic one just has you performing a typical squat where your back is straight and you bend your knees into a squat position, and your kettlebell weight hangs from your arms between your legs, dipping down toward the floor.

Other squat exercises include lowering yourself down while keeping the kettlebell level with your shoulder and the full squat, which lowers you all the way past a sitting position where you're resting on your heels, and you extend the kettlebell overhead until your arms are in a locked position. Other kettlebell movements will originate from your squatting movements.

A swing in the kettlebell world is when you bend over and put the kettlebell between your feet and you start the movement by pushing the bell behind you as if you're spiking a football. Then you pull the bell forward back through your legs and out in front of you as you rise into a standing position.

When you perform a snatch, you are doing the same movement as a swing, only the final position will be where the kettlebell is raised completely overhead. Because the bell has a tendency to flip over and hit your wrist, you need to learn how to control the handle so that you can maneuver it a better position.

The kettlebell clean is another popular movement. For this one, you'll again start out with the bell between your feet. You'll bend down to take a hold of it and like the swing and snatch, push the bell behind you, through your legs. Instead of pushing it out and forward or straight up, you'll bring the kettlebell close to your body as if you're doing a curl, but you won't actually be curling it.

These are some of the most basic movements when you're using a kettlebell. When you are researching the more advanced ones, you'll find that the starting positions are almost always one of the ones listed above.

A few will have an unusual starting position, such as the Turkish Get Up, which begins with you lying flat on your back on the floor and finishing in a raised and lunging position.

Top Kettlebell Movements For Complete Home Workouts

The kettlebell is often heralded as a fantastic training tool thanks to its ability to train the body in a less conventional manner that involves more of our supporting muscle groups and challenges balance and focus at the same time.

This is only one advantage of the kettlebell though. What's just as impressive is just how versatile the tool is – allowing you to train every muscle group in a vast variety of different ways. In fact, a kettlebell is versatile enough to provide an entire body workout and can be a 'home gym' all on its own!

Here are some kettlebell movements that demonstrate this nicely:

Kettlebell Curl

The kettlebell curl is a movement that works similarly to a regular curl and targets the biceps. The difference is that the center of gravity is lower down, thereby altering the angle and changing the direction of the force.

Goblet Squat

Something that is very hard to do when training from a home gym is work the legs using squatting motions. Squats are widely regarded as some of *the* most functional movements and are particularly popular thanks to their ability to engage lots of large muscles in the posterior chain. The problem is that they require a large, heavy and unwieldy squat rack and bar! Or do they?

Using a kettlebell, you can hold the weight against your chest and then squat from there. This moves the weight forward slightly but is otherwise effectively the same movement as any other squat!

Straight Legged Deadlift

The deadlift is another movement lacking from most home workouts and once again, the kettlebell comes to the rescue. A deadlift can be performed as normal, simply by squatting and grabbing the handle with both hands.

Likewise though, you can also train similarly while keeping both legs straight and bending only at the back to hit the erector spinae. This works better considering the slightly lighter and taller nature of a kettlebell.

Turkish Get Up

Now for something *entirely* unique. The Turkish get-up is a movement that requires you to lie on the floor next to your kettlebell and then simply stand up with it. This is much harder than it sounds and involves a complex sequence of movements that train the muscles in unison.

Kettlebell Swing

This is perhaps the king of kettlebell movements and involves performing a squat like motion while swinging the kettlebell behind yourself between your legs and then up in front of yourself. The key is to use a continuous motion and to use your hips to thrust the weight forward rather than engaging your legs or back too much.

Kettlebell Clean and Press

This movement is good in all kinds of ways and involves squatting down to grab a kettlebell in one hand, then throwing it up to lean against the shoulder, standing up and pressing it over head. This trains a huge range of different movements but what's perhaps most effective of all about it is that you are training on just one side of the body – meaning you need to work *very* hard to maintain balance and to stabilize yourself.

Kettlebell Drills You Can Do at Home

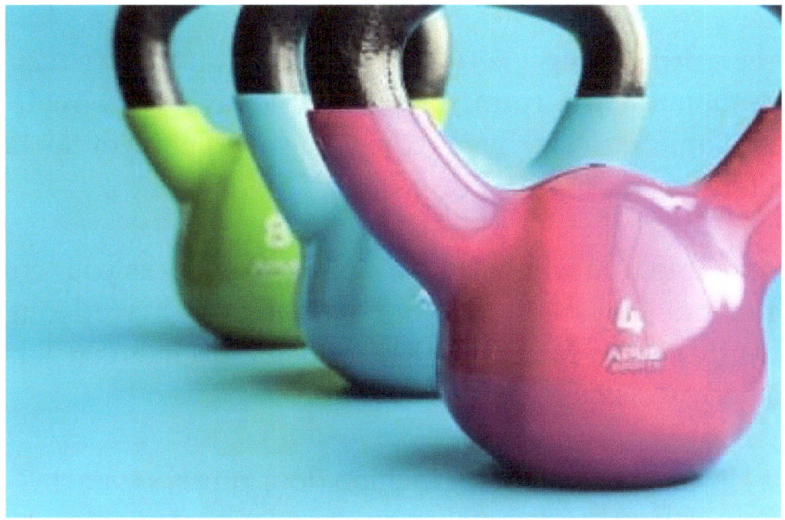

Kettlebells can be used anywhere – in a gym, indoors or outdoors. Many people prefer to do kettlebell drills at home and create a combination of movements or drills that maximize their workouts.

In a gym, you've probably seen circuit training set ups where you move from one machine to the next, keeping your heart rate up with short breaks in between of a few seconds.

This is a wonderful way to include aerobic training in your day. But it also allows you to put a focus on resistance training at the same time – one of the perks of using kettlebells as your primary fitness equipment.

Set up your own circuit course in your home with your kettlebell exercises. They're generally only done for up to one minute total, but some people increase that to two minutes if they want more reps.

Exercise drills using a kettlebell will help you achieve results faster than a slower routine. You want to give your circuit course some variety when it comes to which parts of the body it will focus on.

For example, you will have one station that works your core, another one that spotlights your legs, and one to work out your upper body. Many of the kettlebell movements will be total body workouts, too.

Your circuit training might include floor presses for arms and legs, swings and snatches or clean up movements. Combine several movements to create a drill of your own. For example, you might combine a 1 arm snatch with an overhead squat.

You could implement a kettlebell drill scenario where you have an isolation circuit. This is where, instead of working out multiple areas of your body, you'll focus on one muscle or area at a time.

For example, one of your circuit stops in your home could be the kettlebell curl. This would specifically work out your biceps and wouldn't have a strong impact on your core or the trunk of your body.

The key is to switch up your kettlebell drills and ensure your body is receiving a good variety of exercises. You also want to vary your routine so that you're not overworking one area and possibly creating a situation where injury can occur.

Keep the exercise routine fun for you. If there's one kettlebell drill that you despise, see if you can find one that works out the same area of your body, but does it in a way that you enjoy.

Kettlebell DVD Training

You don't need to join a group class or try to perform a kettlebell routine on your own without proper guidance. All you need to do is pop in a kettlebell DVD and you can have private training right in the comfort of your own home.

Just as you would do with an in-person class, make sure you find a DVD for your correct level of training. If you've never tried using kettlebells, make sure you start with a beginner's DVD.

Many of the DVDs will have a variety of levels for you to choose from. So you might start out on the beginner's level, but then forward to the medium and advanced levels on the same DVD when you're ready.

Some of the kettlebell DVDs will have a short routine that you simply repeat for the duration of your workout. For example, it might be a 15-minute training session that you repeat four times for an hour workout. Then it might include a longer workout for those who want more variety.

People get very picky about fitness DVDs. You might not like the sound of the person's voice or feel they talk too much (or too little). It could irritate you if the participants are smiling non-sop, or if they're stick-thin and don't represent the masses watching the DVD to lose weight.

Make sure you review all of these little idiosyncrasies before you invest in a set of DVDs for your kettlebell training efforts. Find out what the music is like, too – if that's an important element for you.

Your kettlebell DVD should have a warm-up and cool down routine. Usually, the warm up routine is created where the instructor is walking you through the various moves you're about to do in the higher intensity portions, but at a slower pace.

You might find that some of the moves are too difficult for you to do on the DVD. If this happens, continue training on the parts you can do and each time you turn on the DVD again, attempt the exercise that was previously an obstacle for you. Eventually you'll discover that you're able to do it because your strength has increased.

Because the kettlebell originated from Russia, you will see many DVDs presented by a Russian persona. This could be inspiring for you or wear thin if you dislike overuse of the word comrade.

Once you find a trainer that meshes well with your personality, look for the right DVD that has a bunch of different workout for you and ample safety and proper form instructions.

Kettlebell Workout Tips

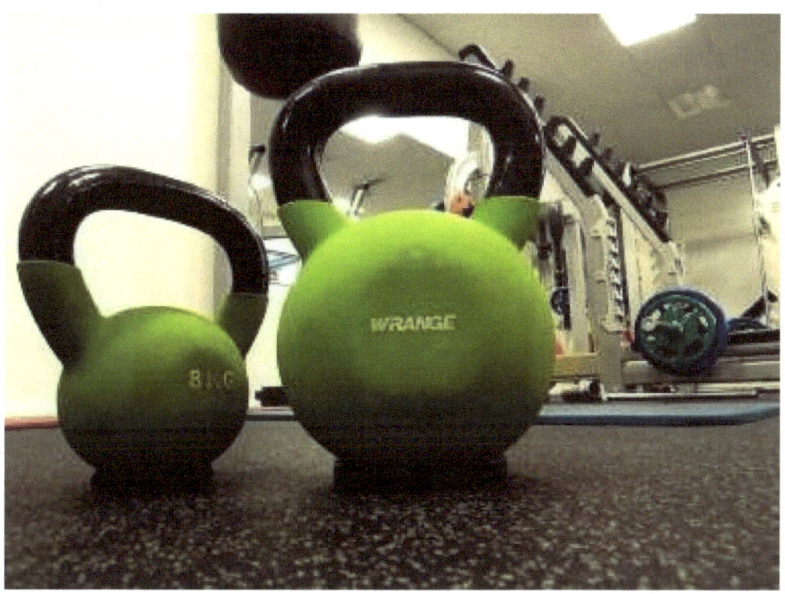

The main thing you want to do when preparing for a kettlebell workout is to have safety in mind before you get started. That's the rule with any fitness program – if you are putting stress on your body, you want to do it the right way or you risk injury.

With kettlebells, you're working with a heavy piece of equipment (usually made of cast iron), and pair that with the many swinging or high speed movements and you have a recipe for disaster if you haven't considered the safety aspect.

Make sure you have plenty of room to perform the exercises. You don't want to swing a kettlebell and accidentally put a hole in your wall. Slowly move the kettlebell around in all directions to make sure you have plenty of room without the risk of hitting something.

Kettlebell workouts range from basic beginner moves to more advanced strategies. Start with a good foundation in understanding the routines and then escalate your workout to something more.

Because you'll be holding these weights with your hands and moving them rapidly, you don't want sweaty palms to cause you to lose control of the kettlebell. Keep the dampness minimized by using a towel frequently – or by wearing workout gloves to help you keep your grip.

Look to a professional for the best kettlebell workout tips. You can take a local class, buy a DVD or even read and see instructions online to help you maneuver the workouts, but instructions are necessary to prevent injury and help you reach your fitness goals.

When you start your training, make sure you begin with a weight that's manageable for you. Don't overdo it and start with a kettlebell that's too heavy because it will actually do more harm than good.

It's best to have a set of kettlebells where you can change up the weight according to the movement. Some movements may require more repetition and lighter weight, while other slower exercises would be perfect with a heavier weight.

Make sure you rest between sets. You don't want to cause injury or burn out before your workout is complete. You want to vary the routines you tackle, too. Doing the exact same movements over and over again means your body isn't getting the benefit of what the kettlebells can do for you.

You can even alter an exercise slightly to get more out of it. For example, slowing a ballistic movement down to a grinding movement (fast to slow) can help improve your strength and assist you in building a formidable core.

The Hidden Crucial Factor in Kettlebell Training: Grip Strength

If you want to become amazing at kettlebell training, then there is one thing you need to develop more than anything else and that is *grip strength*. A firm and powerful grip is precisely what will enable you to lift heavier kettlebells for longer periods of time, not to mention the best way to ensure that you don't accidentally launch them through the window in your local gym...

Meanwhile though, building amazing grip strength will benefit you in areas that extend far beyond the reaches of the kettlebell and this is actually one of the biggest reasons *to* take up this kind of training in the first place. By taking up kettlebell training, you'll be able to build forearm and grip power that will translate to improved performance in just about every aspect of your life.

The question then becomes: how do you develop the kind of grip strength that you need for kettlebell training? And why is it so important anyway?

Why Grip Strength is Crucial

If you want to improve your performance on *any* movement in the gym, then training your grip strength is essential. Grip strength gives you a firmer hold on the bar or weight and this in turn means that more of the force you apply will go into the *movement* rather than just holding onto the weight. This can also help you to last longer on movements like pull ups or deadlifts before fatiguing.

This is something that old-time strongmen knew very well and hence they would train with weights that had wider bars for instance in order to increase the challenge for their grip. This also prevented anyone from their audience from stepping up and showing them up by being able to lift the same weights. No matter how strong they were, they would normally lack that crucial grip strength.

And in the real world, grip strength is useful for: opening jam jars, combat, climbing, using tools, carrying luggage and more!

How to Develop Grip Strength

Training with kettlebells is one excellent way to develop grip strength because the weights swing. Each time you perform one of the movements, the angle will change, forcing you to tighten your grip in response and thereby keep the weights held firmly rather than dropping.

There are many more ways you can develop grip strength though in your training and these will help you to improve your kettlebell workouts as well as many other aspects of your training.

Good examples include:
- Performing pull ups by gripping onto a rope or even a towel looped over a pull up bar
- Performing curls with thicker bars
- Training using a grip trainer
- Attempting to bend bars
- Performing wrist curls and other exercises that specifically target forearms

Another great option is taking up rock climbing and in particular, traversing. Rock climbing requires you to hold onto the small holes and jutting out rocks that you can grip onto. Traversing means climbing *along* the wall instead of up and this is an ideal form of exercise as it allows you to climb without a rope (you never get more than a meter off the ground) and means you are gripping onto the wall for longer periods of time while you find your footing.

What to Expect in Kettlebell Classes

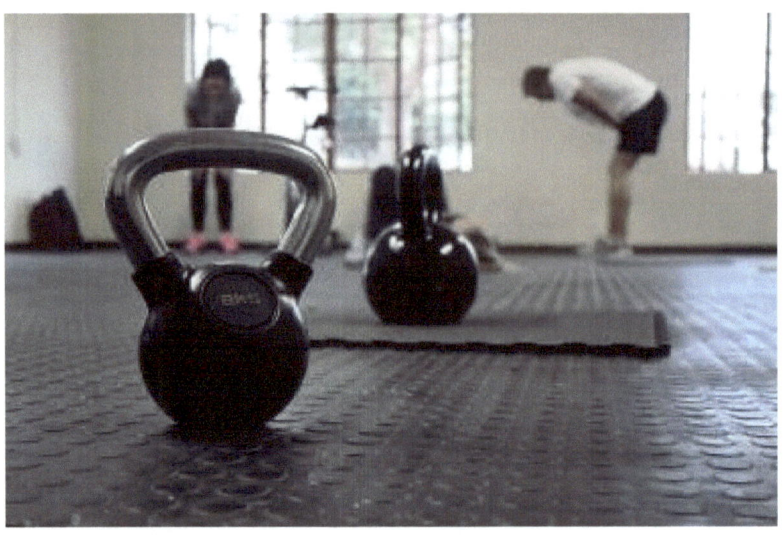

Kettlebell classes can be found in almost any larger city, and some smaller areas, too. As with any fitness class, you're going to find instructors who suit your needs, those that are too advanced, and some who fall behind what your body is capable of handling.

You can find kettlebell classes that are just for women, just for men, or a combination of genders. They're usually limited in numbers, since each person will need ample space to swing and move with the kettlebell.

If you're new to kettlebell training, then you'll want to start out by finding a beginner's class. This type of class will show you the proper form in handling kettlebells and the right way to pick up the equipment and maneuver it to prevent injury and maximize your workout.

Most classes last about an hour, and in some cases, you may be required to have completed a specific level of training in another class before you sign up for a more advanced class.

There's usually not a lot of talking in these types of fitness classes because the repetition and speed of the training means everyone is concentrating on his or her own workout and paying attention to their form.

Prepare to sweat a lot in a kettlebell class, so take a gym towel with you. This will prevent you from getting drenched, but it can also help you maintain control over the kettlebell, since sweaty hands could send the equipment flying through the air if you lose your grip.

Some classes will ask you to bring your own kettlebells – or you might simply have a preference for your own equipment. Other classes will provide a set of kettlebells for each person in attendance, so that you can choose the weight that's right for you.

Many local kettlebell classes keep their groups small in nature so that more personal attention is given to every participant. You may prefer this or the anonymity of a larger class.

Try to find a kettlebell class where the instructor switches up the routine every day. You want someone who is innovative in his or her thinking about this type of exercise, so that boredom never sets in.

There are also specific kettlebell classes for rehabilitation, if you've been injured and need to use this form of exercise to help rebuild your strength and fitness stamina.

There are even classes created for tactical career individuals, such as police, military and firefighters.

Kettlebell for Women

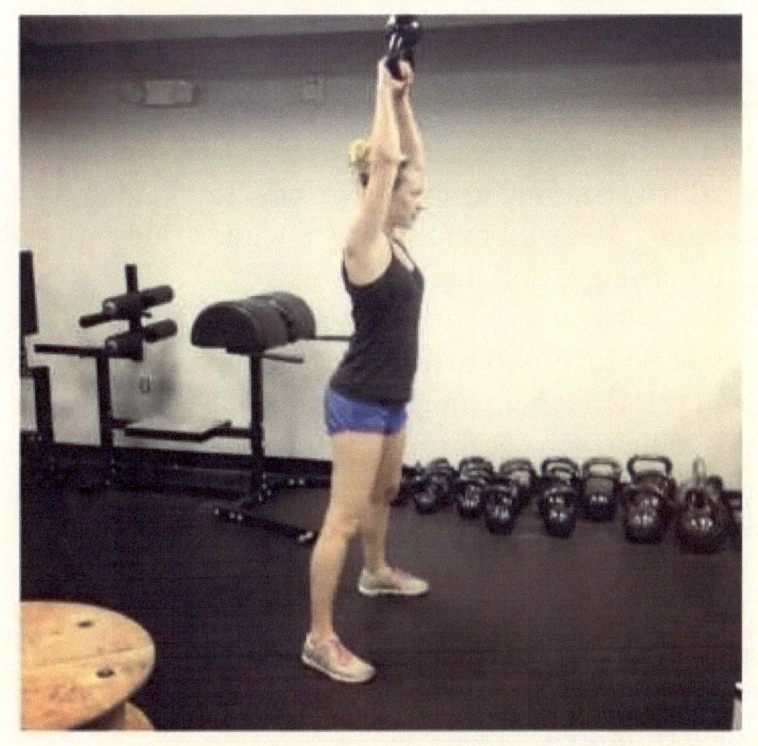

Men and women have different bodies, so expecting the same workout routine or equipment to have identical results isn't feasible. We often want different results, anyway. Men like to bulk up and get lean, while women often want to slim down and firm up.

Choosing kettlebell for women means you're going to be picking a different set of the kettlebells themselves. You'll probably be choosing a separate workout DVD for kettlebell training. And your routines won't be the same as it would be for men who are bodybuilding.

You'll find specific kettlebell for women training by all of the top fitness names like Jillian Michaels, Bob Harper, Pavel Tsatsouline, and Kathy Smith. These will walk you through the routines you need to get in shape.

There are some kettlebell for women DVDs that focus on fat loss and cardio. You can expect these routines to include more ballistic training instead of grinds. Remember ballistic means it includes a lot of movement, while grinds are slow-paced for strength building.

You might be surprised to know that there are kettlebell for women DVDs that help pregnant women. You can use a DVD like this to help you get through your pregnancy in a fit way, but also to recover your pre-pregnancy body after you deliver.

Because many women have busy lives, you'll be happy to know that there are kettlebell training sessions that can be done in short increments. For example, you'll find 6-minute kettlebell training DVDs for women.

There are many ways that women benefit from the use of kettlebells. Fat loss is the primary reason many women engage in this type of training. But that's not the only thing it can do.

Kettlebells also help you build strong bones and assist you in training your joints to function better. It provides a method of strength training without the unwanted side effect of bulking up in mass.

Many women have turned to kettlebell training. They range from top athletes to celebrities, from CEOs to housewives and even senior citizens have latched onto the kettlebell craze. Runners who are already lean have begun to adopt the kettlebell regimen because it assists them in increasing their endurance for marathons and races.

Many women have reported that kettlebell training has given them a certain amount of power in their everyday lives. They no longer need help carrying heavy objects or opening jars that previously required more upper body strength than they could muster. Now, they have a whole new body, ready to take on anything at any time.

Buying a Kettlebell

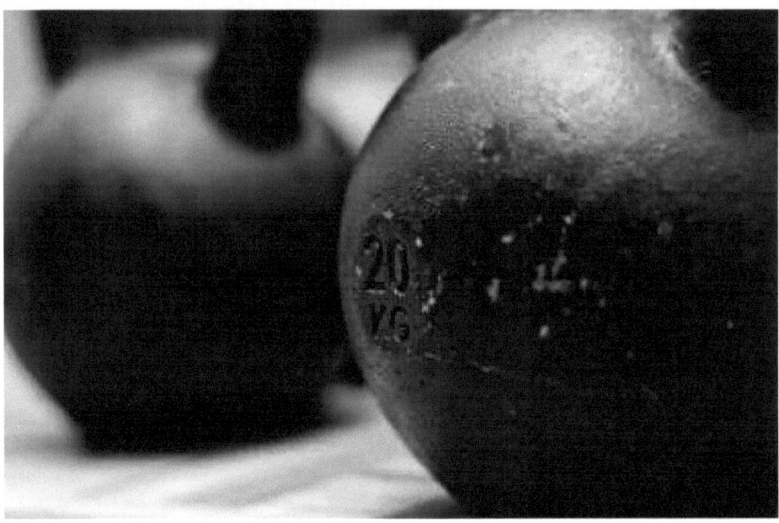

There are many reasons you might want to buy a kettlebell. They burn a lot of fat with their strength training and cardiovascular combination. They're affordable, don't take up a lot of space, and you can get a lot of results with just a little bit of effort.

Kettlebells are very trendy, but they're not the same as a flash in the pan fad. Kettlebells have actually been around for a very long time and have just maintained their reputation as a formidable piece of exercise equipment.

You can buy a kettlebell locally (if you can find them) or online. If you buy online, there are some places that will provide free shipping, which is a perk, considering they're made of heavy cast iron materials in most cases.

There are kettlebells for women and those for men, but in reality, it just depends on how much you can lift and endure during your training routine.

You can buy kettlebells in sets or individually, too.

For many workouts, you'll only need a single kettlebell. But for some routines, you'll be using two kettlebells – one in each hand. This is primarily for the more advanced kettlebell user, not beginners.

Some of the kettlebells that you buy come with more components than just the kettlebells themselves. Some of them come in kits – complete with a DVD, training manual, nutrition guide and workout chart.

You might want to stick with the traditional cast iron kettlebells, but many people are now choosing kettlebells that are made of alternate materials. For example, you might find some that are filled with sand and covered with vinyl so that they won't put marks on your floor like a cast iron version would.

Just make sure that whatever material you invest in, the kettlebell itself resembles the original kettlebell shape, with a handle positioned for you to grip easily and a base that's flat below the rounded part.

Some people prefer to buy a set of kettlebells in many different increments. Others like to buy an adjustable kettlebell. This is where you have one kettlebell, but you can adjust the weight of it in increments.

Kettlebells have an aesthetic appeal, too. Some women like to get a girly color, like pink. Some prefer to invest in a kettlebell that looks powerful and daunting, like one with a skull etched into the rounded part.

There are some kettlebell sets that have stands where you can stack the equipment vertically. However, unless you have a large set of kettlebells, you can store these easily almost anywhere out of sight.

If you are shopping for a kettlebell (a giri or girya in Russian), you probably want to know what different types are available. Can men and women and use the same kettlebell? And what weight should you get? If you have never used a kettlebell before, should you purchase a different type of product than someone who is familiar with the "cannonball with a handle"? And just how did this odd looking cardiovascular, strength and flexibility training device originate? You have questions, and we have all the answers in this definitive guide to buying kettlebells.

What is a kettlebell and where did it come from?

Kettlebells date back to the 1700s in Russia. A large, round cast-iron or steel weight with a handle, kettlebells facilitate swinging and ballistic movements. They were not used for exercise originally. Rather, farmers used them to weigh crops. At markets and festivals were they sold their goods, these farmers enjoyed showing off the strength they had developed from constantly lifting these heavy weights.

The Soviet Army began using them as physical training and conditioning equipment in the 20th century, and sports competition began in Russia and Europe in the 1940s. Kettlebells became popular as a strength and cardio training device in the United States in the 1960s, and are now found in health and fitness clubs throughout the country .

What types of kettlebells can I choose from?

You will find some sand-filled kettlebells on the market and even a few filled with water, but generally they are made from either professional grade steel or standard grade cast-iron.

Cast-iron

When choosing cast-iron, the larger the bell size, the heavier the weight. The smaller the bell size, the lower the weight. There may be a slight difference in handle diameter and width as well. The handle will be thicker than on competition steel bells, and may not be best for people with small hands. Cast-iron kettlebells will almost always be less expensive.

Steel

Competition bells, made of high-grade steel, are always the same size. They will vary in weight, but the size is uniform to guarantee a standard lifting technique. Competition steel kettlebells are always more expensive than cast-iron, since they must adhere to national and international competition specifications. The handles on steel kettlebells are thinner than their cast-iron counterparts, and are specially designed to prevent slipping.

Whether beginner or veteran weight trainer, what should I be looking for?

Beginning weight trainer

You should probably get started with a cast-iron kettlebell as a beginner. Because of their unique design and effect on your body, kettlebells are not for everyone. A cast-iron investment is less expenses, and if you find out you enjoy the intense, one-of-a-kind kettlebell training exercises and benefits, you can always step up to the more expensive, professionally constructed competition bells.

However, if you have the money to invest in competition grade kettlebells from the start it is highly recommended that you do so. The handles are thinner and easier to grasp, slip-free design is integrated, and the ball portion of the device is always the same size, regardless what weight bell you purchase.

Veteran weight trainer

You will probably want to get started immediately with competition steel kettlebells. As a veteran weight trainer, you understand the importance of form over function. Steel kettlebells allow for a perfect and consistent range of motion for each repetition. And when you get stronger and move up to a heavier weight, the uniform size and easy grip handle mean you will continue to practice perfect form. Proper form delivers quicker results and fewer injuries, whenever weight training is involved.

Should men and women use different sized weights, and what weight size is best for me?

Men and women should first choose bells according to the above criteria. As far as weight is concerned, women probably want to start off with an 8 kg or 10 kg bell (15 or 20 pound sizes are comparable in the US). Men should probably start with a 12 kg to 16 kilogram bell (roughly 25 to 35 pound US equivalent). Not sure what weight is right for you? Choose the lighter weight above, or find a local gymnasium or health club which uses kettlebells and get some hands-on experience.

What are some typical kettlebell weights?

Russian kettlebells are usually measured in weight by "poods". 1 pood equals about 16 kilograms (around 35 pounds). In the United States, typical kettlebell weights will range from 10 to 80 or more pounds. This includes both cast-iron and steel competition bells.

In the United Kingdom and other non-US areas, you can expect to find bells beginning as light as 5 kilograms and as heavy as 32 or 36 kilograms. (Remember to always err on the side of caution, and choose the lighter bell when deciding between 2 different weight sizes.)

What exercises can I perform with my kettlebell?

The most common kettlebell exercises are swings, cleans, windmills, and snatches. Single arm swings and 2 arm rows are popular, as are the goblet squat, figure 8 and the Russian twist. There are plenty of videos and instructional e-books available online which walk you through performing each and every kettlebell exercise properly.

What physical benefits do kettlebells deliver?

Moving from the farmer's fields to the Russian Red Army, kettlebells provide an intense total body workout. Because swinging motions are involved, your agility and balance are improved. Obviously lifting weights builds your strength, but your endurance is boosted as well. When done properly and in high repetitions, kettlebell exercises offer improved cardiovascular health and functioning. Your hips, glutes, hamstrings and waistline also benefit from this unique physical fitness tool.

Unlike the more common dumbbell which is also used for single arm weightlifting, kettlebells have a center of mass which moves far beyond your hand. This impacts your body in a greater manner than a dumbbell, involving more muscle groups. Known as an "unstable force" in weight training, this is the primary reason for the greater impact kettlebell training has on your body than standard free weights.

How much do kettlebells cost?

A quick search on Amazon shows that you can purchase a 5 pound kettlebell for around $5. Obviously, you have a shipping charge to consider as well. And that particular price is for a cast-iron bell with a one-piece cast. 25 pound cast-iron kettlebells will be anywhere between $20 and $30 usually, with a 55 pound kettlebell costing between $45 and $55.

Because of their painstaking production and competition level specifications, steel kettlebells are more expensive. 8 kg (15 to 20 pound) models can run as much as $40 online, with a 32 kg (70 pound) professional grade competition kettlebell setting you back $150 or more.

More points to consider

Kettlebells are extremely unique, in both design and exercise. Do not assume that just because you are physically fit that you can start off with a heavy weight. Swinging, snatching and jerking movements need to be perfected before you move up in weight.

You get what you pay for. Cast-iron kettlebells are definitely recommended if you are just getting started. Just remember that uneven bottoms, welded handles, a rough handle finish and sometimes minimal handle clearance can be negatives encountered with the cast-iron version of this product.

It is not always easy to find kettlebells locally. The Internet provides a great place to comparison shop, you will always find exactly what you are looking for, and get delivery right to your front door.

Top 5 Kettlebells Reviewed & Compared

Listed below you will find the top 5 kettlebells sold on Amazon, perfect for both men and women. We took into account company reputation, quality of product, availability, kettlebell type, previous purchaser customer satisfaction rating and weight range. You will also see a price range listed.

Prices and availability may vary according to supply and demand and other factors, but these particular kettlebells consistently rank as the bestselling and highest rated on all of Amazon.

Cast-iron bells are less expensive and perfect for all kettlebell exercises, but are not sanctioned for competition. Competition steel bells are more expensive and of a higher quality, and we designate which type of bells are reviewed below.

1 - Cap Barbell Kettlebell (non-competition grade)

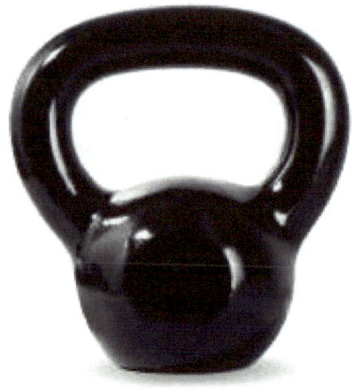

Bell type - Cast-iron
Price range - $25 to $110
Weight range - 15 lb to 80 lb
Amazon customer rating - 4.5 / 5.0 stars
Amazon link: http://amzn.to/2lo7IJs

Since their launch in 1982, Cap Barbell has been creating more than 600 products in 10 weight and physical fitness training categories. Their kettlebells range in size from 15 pounds to 80 pounds, and are made of solid cast iron with a black machine finish. Available for purchase online, all Cap Barbell kettlebells come with a 30 day manufacturers warranty. The handles have been reinforced with steel for durability.

Consistently the bestselling product in the entire kettlebell category at Amazon, these bells are perfect for beginners and veterans. As with all cast-iron bells, size increases with weight. Compared to their cast-iron counterparts, Cap Barbell kettlebells have a smooth finish. This diminishes the risk of chafing and scratching due to frequent use. These make an excellent investment with a mid-range price tag for the beginner to intermediate kettlebell user.

2 - SPRI Deluxe Vinyl Kettlebells (non-competition grade)

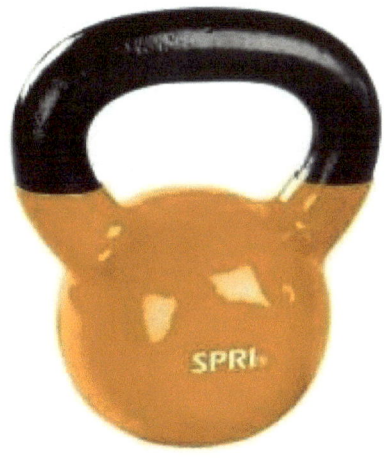

Bell type - Cast-iron
Price range - $16 to $88
Weight range - 5 lb to 50 lb
Amazon customer rating - 4.4 / 5.0 stars
Amazon link: http://amzn.to/2lo3SAa

SPRI specializes in distributing rubberized resistance exercise products. Their kettlebells are color-coded for quick and easy identification of weight size. The company's cast-iron bells are vinyl coated for easier handling, and that coating also means protecting your floors against scratching and other damage.

If you are shopping for kettlebells that deliver a great mix of value and quality, SPRI Deluxe Vinyl Kettlebells are an excellent choice. Consistently a top 10 bestseller on Amazon.

3 - Solid Cast Iron Kettlebell (non-competition grade from Yes4All and other manufacturers)

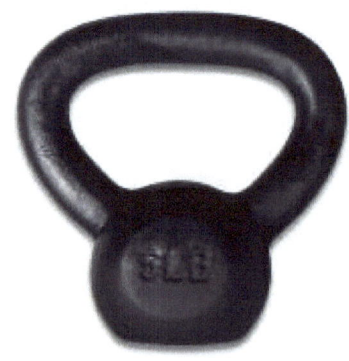

Bell type - Cast-iron
Price range - $5 to $47
Weight range - 5 lb to 60 lb
Amazon customer rating - 4.6 / 5.0 stars
Amazon link: http://amzn.to/2jH8oUw

Perfect for beginners and those who do not want to invest a lot of money before they decide if kettlebell exercising is right for them, these solid cast-iron bells are extremely attractive financially. Offered in 12 different weights and including a rough textured wide handle, these bells have no vinyl finish.

Fewer expensive features keep your costs down. These kettlebells are still perfect for improving your strength, cardiovascular health, balance and agility, while also requiring a minimal financial outlay. Consistently a top 5 bestseller among all kettlebells on Amazon due to the low price.

4 - Body Solid KBS105 5 to 30-Pound Kettle Bell Set (non-competition)

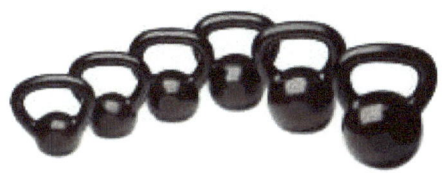

Bell type - Cast-iron
Price range - around $150
Weight range - 5 lb to 30 lb set
Amazon customer rating - 4.7 / 5.0 stars
Amazon link: http://amzn.to/2k3UTQD

Body Solid has created a value based kettlebell set with some nice features. Instead of rough, unfinished cast-iron, these bells are coated with a tough enamel finish. Steel reinforced for excellent durability, this 6 piece set includes 5, 10, 15, 20, 25 and 30 pound bells.

Buying the entire set makes for a less expensive investment than piecing together several purchases. And this attractively priced kettlebell set is accompanied by a limited lifetime manufacturer's warranty. Perfect for the beginner to intermediate user, both male and female.

5 - CFF 16 kg Pro Competition Russian Kettlebell Girya (competition grade)

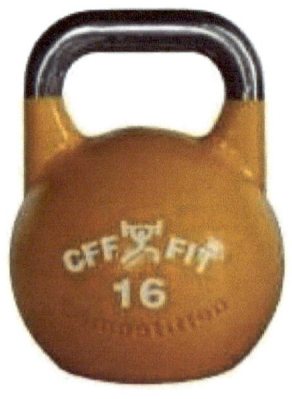

Bell type - Steel
Price range - $45 to $155
Weight range - 8 kg to 32 kg
Amazon customer rating - 4.8 / 5.0 stars
Amazon link: http://amzn.to/2kweKJ5

There is a very good reason that the Pro Competition Russian Kettlebell line of products released by Christian Fitness Factory are rated so high by previous purchasers. Customers who bought these bells through Amazon online frequently award them with perfect 5.0 customer satisfaction ratings. The average rating for the different competition level weight size kettlebells released by CFF is a nearly perfect 4.8 / 5.0 stars.

One piece all steel construction means no possible chipping and cracking as with entry-level cast-iron bells. The CFF bells are also designed with a flat bottom. This makes them perfect for renegade rows and other similar exercises. Weight sizes vary from 8 to 32 kg, with every weight accompanied by a regulation 33 mm handle. This prevents slippage and minimizes fatigue, and is a competition requirement. CFF has color-coded their kettle bells for quick and easy identification by weight size. Definitely a top tier product you need to consider if you are entering kettlebell competitions, or if you just want a top kettlebell product for your own use.

Kettlebell Reviews

If you're new to the kettlebell craze and wondering if you should use them and what type of workout is right for you, then you're going to have to wade through a lot of kettlebell reviews from people with specific tastes in fitness instruction and equipment.

Kettlebell equipment will have people disagreeing in their reviews a lot. You'll find loyal fans of the traditional cast iron equipment and those who prefer sand-filled options that are less destructive to your floor.

So reviewers will suggest that you opt for an entire set of kettlebells, while others say one is all you need. There are also some enthusiasts who admire the adjustable kettlebells, so their reviews will all be skewed to personal preferences.

Even color choice and appearances of the kettlebell equipment will have differing reviews. Some like a solid black kettlebell, like they used in Russia in traditional times, while others appreciate the multi-colored sets or those with carvings that suggest power and strength.

Kettlebell classes that you can take locally will sometimes have reviews online. You want to listen to what people are saying about the instructor, the limits on the number of participants, and the variety in the routines themselves.

You might ask to attend a single class for free (most gyms will allow this one time) to see if you and the instructor are a good fit for one another. Sometimes it's not the trainer at all but the group of people who will sway you to like or dislike the class.

Kettlebell DVDs have a wide range of reviews. You'd be amazed at how many quirks irritate people when they repeatedly watch a kettlebell DVD day after day. You may or may not agree with the reviews that you read, so you might want to find a segment of the instructor on YouTube or elsewhere to see if you like them.

Some of the things that most bother kettlebell DVD reviewers are the background music, the style or frequency of the instructor's voice appearing in the workout, the body types of the participants in the background, and even the fact that some of them may smile too much!

Many of those little things may not bother you at all, so you have to take the star ratings with a grain of salt and dig into the written reviews a bit more to see if the reviewer is just being too picky.

Kettlebell routines can be reviewed online. You have so many options with kettlebell routines. You can mix the grinds and ballistic movements up into a myriad of combinations, and some of them have great feedback while others (such as those hard on the knees) are decimated online.

How to Lose Weight With a Kettlebell

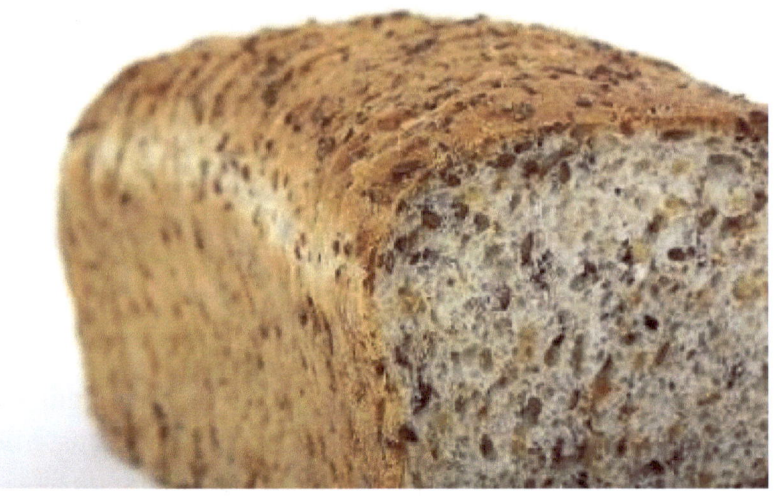

Kettlebell training has a large number of different advantages and lets you train your body from different angles and in a far more functional range of motion.

But what's really great about the kettlebell is versatile it is as a tool and how it allows you develop your fitness and health in numerous different ways.

If you want to build bodybuilder-type muscle, then you can do so by using single joint isolation movements and heavy resistance. This will create muscle fiber tears, flood your muscles with metabolites and generally help you to encourage more growth.

At the same time though, you can also use a kettlebell to lose weight and it happens to be particularly well suited to that goal. Let's look at how you might do that...

The Exercises

The great thing about the kettlebell is that it allows you to perform resistance cardio. This means you are using cardiovascular training that increases your heartrate and helps you to burn fat.

At the same time though, you are also lifting weight, which protects your muscle from breakdown and increases the challenge, thereby increasing the amount of calories burned and the amount of effort involved.

Also useful, is that the kettlebell allows you to train in this manner on the spot and without a lot of tools. Unlike running, you can enjoy kettlebell training in any *weather* and in a short space of time.

And to get the very most of this, you can combine the kettlebell as a tool with the HIIT modality. HIIT is 'high intensity interval training' – a form of exercise that challenges you to alternate between brief bursts of high intensity exertion and shorter periods of relatively steady-state exercise.

In this case for example, you might perform the kettlebell swing for 1 minute and then rest for 30 seconds before going again.

The kettlebell swing is an ideal movement for resistance cardio that involves swinging the kettlebell between your legs and then straight back up in the air using a slight hip thrust movement to provide the forward momentum.

The Diet
To lose weight, this training must be combined with the right type of diet.

That diet should be one that is relatively low in calories. The objective here is to burn more calories in a day than you consume. So if you normally burn 2,000 calories and consume 2,200 calories, you can increase that burn to 2,400 using HIIT training and you can then reduce the amount you eat to 2,100 calories. Now you're losing 300 calories every day!

Try to eat more protein and you will support more muscle growth while reducing fat storage. Combine this with 4 workouts a week, lasting about 20 minutes each and you should start to see the results you're looking for using just this one tool and one movement.

Remember though, weight loss is only achievable if you change your entire lifestyle and habits. It is not enough to simply add in an exercise and forget about it! Walk more, spend less time in front of the TV and reduce unhealthy snacks!

The Forgotten Muscle Groups That Kettlebell Training Works

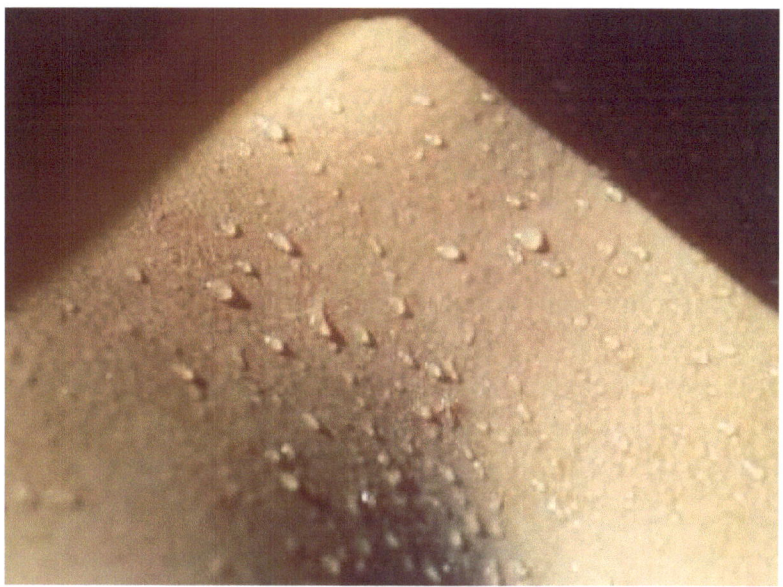

In the last few years, the 'gym bro' has become an anachronism. Old ideas about strength training are falling by the wayside and more and more, we are experimenting with alternative techniques that ultimately present greater benefits in and out of the gym.

So what is a gym bro? What are these old approaches that have fallen out of favor?

The Problem With Old Fashioned Training Ideas

Chief among the ideas that are moving aside is the focus on the 'mirror muscles'. Your typical gym rat in the 00's was obsessed with the idea of building bigger biceps, bigger pecs and toned abs and had little regard for smaller supportive muscles that helped to develop true 'functional strength' that translated to actual performance improvements and better health.

If you train only some muscles at the expense of others, then you will develop an uneven physique that places uneven pressure on your body and ultimately leads to injury.

This is why multi-joint exercises and exercises that force you to move your body through a more dynamic range of motion trainers.

And the kettlebell is the perfect example of more adaptive training methodology...

Why Kettlebell Training is the Solution

When you train with a kettlebell, you are using a weight that is unevenly distributed. That is to say that the center of gravity can move as you move the weight, thereby altering the angle of the resistance and adding new elements like balance and resistance.

This forces you to brace your body and balance yourself in ways you wouldn't have to with something like a bicep curl and that is what allows you to bring in the involvement of your smaller supporting muscles found throughout your body.

So what supporting muscles are you training in particular?

Here are some examples:

Obliques: The obliques are the muscles that run down either side of the abs and are used for bending from side to side and also twisting the torso (applying toque). They are very useful for a range of different movements and are great for aesthetics too – actually making the abs look considerably more impressive.

Serratus Muscles: These muscles are found on the sides of the pecs and are used for extending the arm forward when straight. Again, they can create a more ripped physique and actually provide considerable extra force when engaging in pushing movements.

Forearms: One of the most important muscle groups trained by the kettlebell swing and other movements is the forearms. These include your forearm flexors and extensors which allow you to grip and release things. By improving your grip, you gain a firmer hold on any weight or tool you're training with and thereby greatly improve your performance.

Erector Spinae: These are two muscles trained by the deadlift as well as many other movements. Their job is to help you stand up straight and keep the spine erect. They can help to combat back problems as well as giving you considerably more lifting power!

Final Thoughts

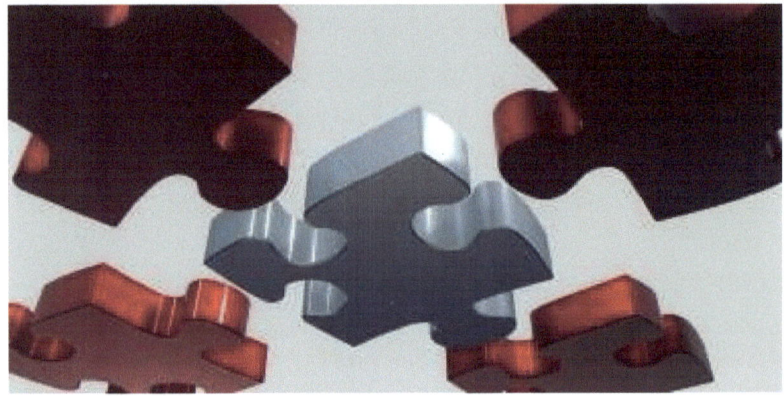

Could kettlebell training be the missing link to your fitness program? If you want to get into a lean, slim, toned and sexy shape, the only tool you're ever going to need to complete this goal is the kettlebell. Let's take a final look at why this is the *perfect* solution for those particular training goals and what you need to do to make it happen.

Enter: Resistance Cardio

The first huge advantage that training with a kettlebell has is that it allows you to use what is known as 'resistance cardio'.

This basically means that you're combining resistance training (this is the term used to describe training that requires muscular force to push or pull a heavy object) with cardio (any exercise that continues for an extended period and thereby gets your heartrate up and helps you burn fat).

By using a movement like the kettlebell swing for 70 repetitions for example, you're going to be forced to lift the weight while also repeating a rapid movement that will mean you have to burn calories stored as fat.

When you combine these two different training modalities, you are building muscle and you are burning fat at the same time. This is great for getting an attractive body because you're not going to simply become skinny (or worse, 'skinny fat').

Rather, resistance cardio will allow you to tone and burn at the same time. The fact that you're engaging muscle means the muscle will be protected from deterioration as you're training.

Moreover, resistance cardio will allow you to burn more fat in a shorter space of time than you could otherwise. This is because you will be forced to apply more effort in order to complete the movement, thereby taxing your system more and burning through more calories!

The Benefits of the Kettlebell Swing

The other great thing about building muscle while performing a cardio workout, is that the more muscle you add, the more you increase your metabolism. If you have lots of muscle, you will burn more calories even while you're sleeping! At the same time, each workout that causes muscle damage will trigger the release of anabolic hormones like testosterone and growth hormone that actually increase the rate of fat loss.

The kettlebell swing is a particularly useful move because it targets the entire posterior chain – the muscles in the legs and back involved in jumping. These are some of the largest muscles in the body and thus this results in a massive flood of hormones and a lot of effort on your part.

And finally, for women who are looking to get toned buttocks and legs, the kettlebell swing is ideal because those are the exact muscles that it trains. This is the same combination of muscles as those used in squatting and if you do a Google search for 'women who squat', you'll see that they are famous for having particularly round and firm glutes. If that's the look you're going for, then there are few moves better than the humble kettlebell swing!

And while you are here, be sure to download our amazing free report *7 Common Kettlebell Workout Mistakes* at: https://secretsofaging.net/wp-content/uploads/2017/01/KettlebellWorkout/KettlebellTransformation/KettlebellMistakes/SqueezePage/index-Edited-New.xht.

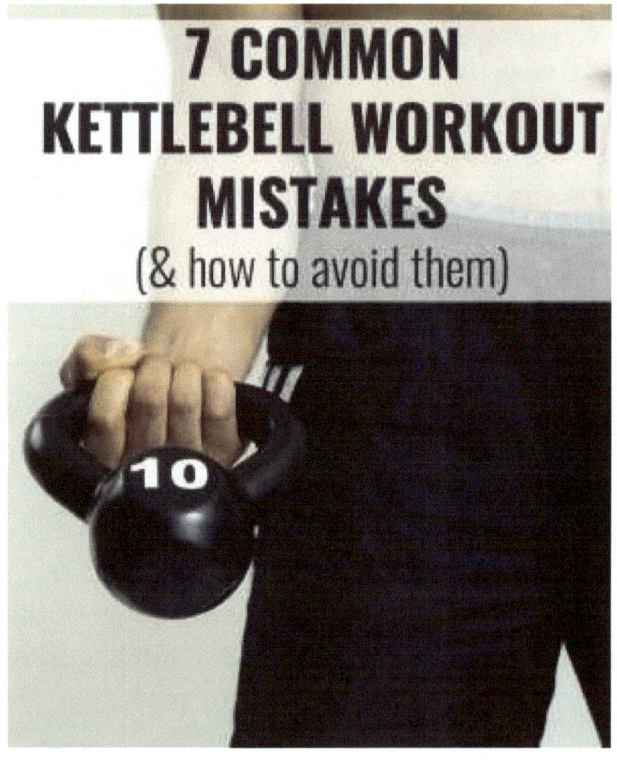

Other Relevant Books by This Author

If you would like to read more relevant books about this topic, here is a list of the CreateSpace links, titles and descriptions from this author:

https://www.createspace.com/6880021

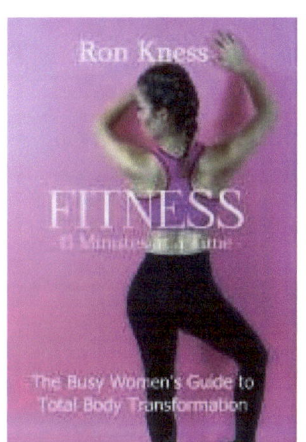

FITNESS - 15 Minutes at a Time: The Busy Women's Guide to Total Body Transformation

We want to be healthier. We also want to be empowered with maintaining our weight and fitness level. And we want to keep the weight off and maintain our healthy lifestyle for the rest of our life!

We can achieve ALL of these goals with the newest release from Ron Kness called "Fitness 15 Minutes at a Time". Based on these exciting teachings, you will learn about all the dramatic benefits of getting fit by eating healthy food resulting in weight loss, and doing high intensity exercising.

This book is built around a very clear, concept: improving your appearance and health.

It's not just about getting healthy. Having great fitness level is linked to reducing the risk of many diseases and even reversing the effects of some, such as being overweight and out of shape. These are just two of the many health benefits of being fit and at a normal weight.

In this book, we look at all the ways you can improve your own fitness level, starting with making the decision to get lose weight and healthy. That is the first step - you must want to do it!

This book also looks at the many other steps that can be taken to support this goal, from creating a calorie deficit - burning more calories than you eat - to exercising at a high intensity, to switching to a fitness and weight maintenance mode once at goal . The choices you make about the kind of food you eat and portion sizes has a big impact on your fitness level.

In "Fitness 15 Minutes at a Time", we'll cover all the bases, giving you everything you need to know to eat healthy, lose weight and get fit.

https://www.createspace.com/6334475

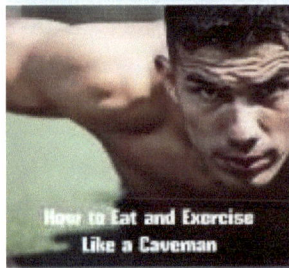

Primal Fitness Fundamentals: How to Eat and Exercise Like a Caveman

In this day of age, we have come a long way compared to the cavemen that once walked our planet. Technology has completely changed our world (and not always for the better when it comes to health and fitness). It has made it easier for us to harvest and gather crops and kill animals for meat. – just go to the grocery store. It has become so advanced that fruits, vegetables and animal products are being mass produced at a large scale to accommodate a huge population of people.

Cavemen used to have to walk and sprint for days (bodyweight exercise) to feed their family and there certainly wasn't enough food to feed outside their clan, or last for more than a couple of days. While this may seem terrible, this kind of activity kept them fit even when not fully fed.

Now that we have all this technology helping us gather our food it has created a negative impact on our population. We have now become sedentary throughout our days and barely even have to get up to make our own food. Instead of hunting for some meat, we drive to our local grocery store, or butcher shop. Instead of picking from fruit trees, we pick it up at the store or even have it delivered to our house. These conveniences, we have created to make our lives easier, have made us motionless, overweight and unhealthy.

In order to combat our now sedentary way of life, we have created gyms that provide a means to fitness but these machines only help us so much. Most of these machines only target specific areas of the body and cause us to do motions our body was not efficiently designed to do. Instead, we should be focusing on primal fitness using compound exercises with just our bodyweight to get us to ultimate health.

Primal fitness, also called caveman fitness, is a combination of movements that your body was designed to do to help develop full body strength and health. It is also called functional fitness as it develops muscles used for everyday tasks. In other words, it is the practice of using your body and what nature has given you to remain fit and healthy. Nature can provide an unlimited amount of resistance and endurance in a way that gyms just cannot deliver.

Cavemen needed to be fit in order to get their food and survive out in the wild. These activities probably included walking for miles, sprinting, crawling, swimming and climbing; to name a few. These examples are all great examples of what primal fitness entails. Now that you do not need to hunt or gather your own food, due to great technological advances, primal fitness can be evolved into a more modern way to mimic these movements.

Paleo devotees are dedicated to the pursuit of health and fitness through a diet free of processed foods, wheat products that bloat and fatigue the body, and filled with energy-yielding foods that power their workouts.

When you view how these workouts and this diet complement each other, you can see how this program could work for you.

https://www.createspace.com/6449992

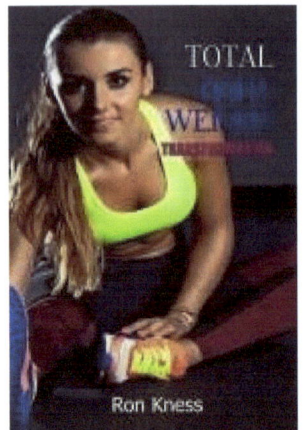

Total Bodyweight Transformation: Discover How to Build Muscle and Burn Fat with No Gyms, Equipment or Complicated Exercises

It's so simple… but bodyweight training might well be the one thing you need to start making some major changes in your life.

Not to say that you necessarily need to be making changes… but if you're looking for a way to build more muscle, to lose fat, to feel healthier and better about yourself and to be pumped full of energy – bodyweight training can do all that.

And this is true even if you have failed to get into shape with other training programs in the past. In fact, bodyweight training is the perfect antidote for anyone who has struggled with regular workouts. Whether you tried running, lifting weights or anything else – bodyweight training presents an answer that is easier, faster and more effective – and that's more likely to help you get the results you're looking for.

Even if you have been successful with other programs in the past – bodyweight training can be the perfect addition to your routine and can help you to get even better benefits even more quickly. And it's a different kind of fitness and strength you'll enjoy too. You'll be strong but you'll also be perfectly proportioned, more full of energy and even more agile.

Bodyweight training gives you power like a coiled spring!

At this point, the first question you might be asking is: why bodyweight training? What's so different about working out with your own body? Why do people succeed with this type of exercise when all else has failed? Let's take a look at some pretty convincing reasons that bodyweight training is what you need…

My book - Total Bodyweight Transformation - has the reasons, exercises and nutrition program you need to get in the best shape of your life.

About the Author

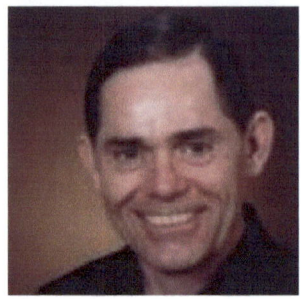

I have published over 125 books on Amazon for Kindle, CreateSpace and other publishing platforms.

While most of my books are on health and fitness in general, as I age (now 65) at the time of this writing) my topics of interest are geared toward aging baby boomers and older.

Besides my own writing, I also ghostwrite ebooks, books, reports, articles, blogs and do Kindle conversions for clients on a variety of topics.

Today my wife and I are retired from our careers and live in Gold Canyon, AZ. I now write as a retirement business where you'll find me happily sitting in my office typing away on my laptop as I work on my next book or ghostwriting project . . . that is if we are not traveling on a cruise ship - our new-found mode of travel.

www.ingramcontent.com/pod-product-compliance
Lightning Source LLC
Chambersburg PA
CBHW040311010626
45792CB00022B/174